BLOOD SUGAR DIET SOLUTION

Burn Fats, Manage Carbohydrates, And Embracing Low-Glycemic Foods With Balanced Meal Planning, Fiber-Rich Breakfast Ideas, Snacks, Physical Activity, And Stress Reduction.

Charlotte Harry

Table of Contents

CHAPTER ONE

UNDERSTANDING BLOOD SUGAR

The Basics Of Blood Sugar

Blood sugar, or glucose, is a fundamental component of your body's energy system. As a simple sugar, it is derived from the foods you consume, primarily carbohydrates. Once you eat, your digestive system breaks down these carbohydrates into glucose, which then enters your bloodstream. This process ensures a steady supply of energy to your cells and organs, allowing them to function optimally. However, the levels of blood sugar can fluctuate based on several factors, including diet, physical activity, and overall health.

The regulation of blood sugar is a vital process managed by your body to maintain homeostasis. Both high and low blood sugar levels can lead to significant health issues. For instance, persistently high blood sugar levels can result in conditions such as hyperglycemia, which is commonly associated with diabetes. On the other hand, low blood sugar levels, known as hypoglycemia, can cause symptoms like dizziness, confusion, and even loss of consciousness if not addressed promptly.

The pancreas, a small yet crucial organ located behind your stomach, plays a significant role in the regulation of blood sugar. It releases hormones that help manage these levels. One of the primary hormones involved is insulin. When you consume food and your blood sugar levels rise, the pancreas releases insulin. Insulin facilitates the uptake of glucose by your cells, where it can be used for energy. It essentially acts as a key, allowing glucose to enter cells and be utilized for various bodily functions.

In addition to insulin, the pancreas also releases glucagon, another hormone that has an opposing effect. When blood sugar levels drop too low, glucagon is released to signal the liver to release stored glucose back into the bloodstream. This balancing act between insulin and glucagon ensures that your blood sugar levels remain within a healthy range.

Diet and lifestyle choices significantly impact blood sugar levels. Consuming a balanced diet rich in whole grains, fruits, vegetables, and lean proteins can help maintain stable blood sugar levels. Regular physical activity also plays a crucial role as it enhances the body's sensitivity to insulin, making it easier for cells to utilize glucose efficiently. Conversely, a diet high in processed foods, sugary drinks, and unhealthy fats can lead to spikes in blood sugar levels and increase the risk of developing insulin resistance.

Overall health also influences blood sugar regulation. Factors such as stress, illness, and hormonal changes can affect how your body manages glucose. Chronic stress, for example, can trigger the release of stress hormones like cortisol, which can raise blood sugar levels. Therefore, managing stress through techniques like meditation, exercise, and adequate sleep is essential for maintaining healthy blood sugar levels.

How Blood Sugar Levels Impact Health

Maintaining balanced blood sugar levels is crucial for overall health and well-being. Blood sugar, or glucose, is the primary source of energy for the body's cells, and its levels are tightly regulated by the hormone insulin, which is produced by the pancreas. When blood sugar levels are too high or too low, it can lead to various health issues that can significantly impact quality of life.

High blood sugar levels, known as hyperglycemia, are commonly associated with diabetes. There are two main types of diabetes: type 1, where the body does not produce insulin, and type 2, where the body does not use insulin properly. Consistently high blood sugar levels can cause damage to blood vessels, which in turn can lead to serious complications such as heart disease, stroke, kidney disease, and nerve damage. These complications arise because excess glucose can cause inflammation and damage to the blood vessels, leading to poor circulation and the buildup of plaque in the arteries.

In addition to the long-term complications, high blood sugar can also cause immediate symptoms such as increased thirst, frequent urination, fatigue, and blurred vision. If left unchecked, hyperglycemia can lead to a dangerous condition called diabetic ketoacidosis, where the body starts breaking down fats at an alarming rate, producing ketones that can make the blood acidic. This condition requires immediate medical attention and can be life-threatening if not treated promptly.

On the other hand, low blood sugar levels, or hypoglycemia, can be equally dangerous. Hypoglycemia occurs when blood glucose levels fall below normal, often as a result of excessive insulin, prolonged fasting, or vigorous exercise. Symptoms of low blood sugar include shakiness, sweating, confusion, irritability, and in severe cases, loss of consciousness. If not promptly addressed, hypoglycemia can lead to seizures and coma. It is crucial for individuals, especially those with diabetes, to monitor their blood sugar levels and have quick sources of glucose available, such as glucose tablets or sugary snacks, to counteract low blood sugar episodes.

Consistently high blood sugar levels can also lead to insulin resistance, a condition where the body's cells become less responsive to insulin. As a result, the pancreas produces more insulin to compensate, which can eventually lead to type 2 diabetes when the pancreas can no longer keep up with the demand. Insulin resistance is often associated with obesity, physical inactivity, and poor dietary habits.

NOTE: To maintain healthy blood sugar levels, it is essential to adopt a balanced diet rich in fiber, whole grains, lean proteins, and healthy fats, while limiting refined sugars and processed foods. Regular physical activity helps improve insulin sensitivity and can aid in maintaining a healthy weight, further reducing the risk of developing diabetes. Additionally, regular monitoring of blood sugar levels, especially for those with diabetes or prediabetes, is vital for early detection and management of blood sugar imbalances.

Symptoms Of High And Low Blood Sugar

Recognizing and understanding the symptoms of high and low blood sugar is crucial for individuals managing diabetes or other blood sugar-related conditions. Prompt action can prevent severe complications and ensure well-being.

Symptoms of High Blood Sugar (Hyperglycemia)

High blood sugar, or hyperglycemia, occurs when there is an excessive amount of glucose in the bloodstream. This condition is often linked to diabetes and can arise from various factors, such as consuming high-sugar foods, lack of insulin, or insufficient physical activity.

Common symptoms of hyperglycemia include:

1.   Frequent Urination: When blood sugar levels are high, the kidneys work harder to filter and remove the excess glucose, leading to increased urination. This symptom is one of the earliest and most noticeable signs.

2.   Increased Thirst: The frequent urination caused by high blood sugar leads to dehydration, prompting the body to crave more fluids. As a result, individuals may experience persistent and intense thirst.

3.   Blurred Vision: Excessive sugar in the blood can cause the lenses of the eyes to swell, resulting in blurred vision. This

symptom can be alarming but is reversible once blood sugar levels are controlled.

4.   Fatigue: High blood sugar levels can interfere with the body's ability to use glucose for energy effectively. Consequently, individuals may feel unusually tired or weak, even after a good night's sleep.

5.   Headaches: Fluctuating blood sugar levels can cause headaches. These headaches can range from mild to severe and may be accompanied by other symptoms such as irritability and difficulty concentrating.

If hyperglycemia is left untreated, it can lead to severe complications like diabetic ketoacidosis (DKA). DKA occurs when the body starts breaking down fats at an alarming rate, producing ketones and making the blood acidic. Symptoms of DKA include nausea, vomiting, abdominal pain, and confusion, and it requires immediate medical attention.

Symptoms of Low Blood Sugar (Hypoglycemia)

Low blood sugar, or hypoglycemia, happens when glucose levels in the blood drop below the normal range. This condition can occur in individuals with diabetes who take insulin or other blood sugar-lowering medications, as well as in those who skip meals or engage in intense physical activity without adequate food intake.

Common symptoms of hypoglycemia include:

1.   Shaking or Trembling: The body's response to low blood sugar is to release adrenaline, which can cause shaking or trembling. This symptom is one of the first signs of hypoglycemia.

2.   Sweating: Increased perspiration is another common sign. Even in a cool environment, individuals experiencing hypoglycemia may break out in a cold sweat.

3.   Rapid Heartbeat: Hypoglycemia triggers the release of stress hormones like adrenaline, leading to a fast or pounding heartbeat.

4.   Dizziness or Lightheadedness: Insufficient glucose in the bloodstream can affect brain function, causing dizziness or a feeling of lightheadedness. This symptom

can be particularly dangerous if it occurs while driving or operating machinery.

5. Hunger: The body's immediate response to low blood sugar is to signal hunger. This intense hunger can come on suddenly and can be difficult to ignore.

6. Irritability or Mood Changes: Low blood sugar levels can impact mood and behavior, leading to irritability, anxiety, or sudden mood swings. These changes can be confusing for both the individual and those around them.

7. Confusion or Difficulty Concentrating: The brain relies heavily on glucose for energy. When blood sugar levels drop too low, cognitive functions can become impaired, resulting in confusion,

difficulty concentrating, or even slurred speech.

NOTE: Understanding these symptoms allows for timely intervention. For hyperglycemia, adjusting medication, increasing physical activity, or modifying diet can help. For hypoglycemia, consuming fast-acting carbohydrates, like glucose tablets or juice, can quickly raise blood sugar levels and alleviate symptoms. By recognizing these signs, individuals can maintain better control over their blood sugar levels and prevent potentially dangerous situations.

The Role Of Insulin

Insulin is a crucial hormone produced by the pancreas that plays a vital role in regulating your body's ability to use and store glucose for energy. When you consume food, especially carbohydrates, your blood sugar levels rise. This increase in blood sugar acts as a signal for the pancreas to release insulin. Insulin facilitates the entry of glucose into your cells, where it can be used immediately for energy or stored for future use, thereby reducing the sugar concentration in your bloodstream.

For individuals with diabetes, the normal production or utilization of insulin is disrupted. There are two main types of diabetes, each affecting insulin differently.

Type 1 Diabetes

In type 1 diabetes, the body's immune system mistakenly attacks and destroys the beta cells in the pancreas that produce insulin. As a result, the pancreas produces little to no insulin. Without sufficient insulin, glucose cannot enter the cells and remains in the bloodstream, leading to high blood sugar levels. People with type 1 diabetes need to take insulin injections or use an insulin pump to manage their blood sugar levels. This exogenous insulin mimics the function of natural insulin, helping to regulate blood sugar by enabling glucose to enter the cells.

Managing type 1 diabetes requires careful monitoring of blood sugar levels, a balanced diet, regular physical activity, and consistent insulin therapy. The goal is to maintain blood sugar levels within a target range to prevent complications associated with high or low blood sugar.

Type 2 Diabetes

Type 2 diabetes, which is more common, involves insulin resistance—a condition where the body's cells do not respond effectively to insulin. Initially, the pancreas compensates for this resistance by producing more insulin. However, over time, the pancreas cannot sustain this increased production, leading to elevated blood sugar levels.

Insulin resistance and type 2 diabetes are often associated with factors such as obesity, sedentary lifestyle, poor diet, and genetics. Unlike type 1 diabetes, type 2 diabetes can often be managed through lifestyle changes, such as a healthy diet and regular exercise. Weight loss and physical activity improve the body's sensitivity to insulin, helping to lower blood sugar levels.

In addition to lifestyle modifications, oral medications that enhance insulin sensitivity or reduce glucose production in the liver are commonly prescribed. In some cases, insulin therapy may also be necessary to achieve adequate blood sugar control.

NOTE: Understanding the role of insulin and how it interacts with glucose in the body is fundamental to managing diabetes. Proper management is crucial to prevent complications such as heart disease, nerve damage, kidney failure, and vision problems. Through a combination of medication, lifestyle changes, and continuous monitoring, individuals with diabetes can lead healthy and active lives.

CHAPTER TWO

THE SCIENCE BEHIND BLOOD SUGAR MANAGEMENT

The Glycemic Index And Glycemic Load

The Glycemic Index (GI) and Glycemic Load (GL) are crucial concepts for understanding how carbohydrates impact blood sugar levels. The Glycemic Index is a numerical scale that ranks carbohydrates based on how quickly they raise blood glucose levels. This scale ranges from 0 to 100, with pure glucose serving as the reference point at 100. High-GI foods, such as white bread and sugary drinks, cause a rapid and significant spike in blood sugar, whereas low-GI foods, like whole grains and vegetables, lead to a more gradual increase in blood sugar.

The GI measures the immediate impact of a carbohydrate-containing food on blood glucose, but it doesn't account for the actual quantity of carbohydrates consumed. This limitation is addressed by Glycemic Load, which combines both the GI of a food and the amount of carbohydrates it contains. By considering both these factors, Glycemic Load offers a more accurate picture of a food's effect on blood sugar levels.

For instance, watermelon has a high Glycemic Index because it can quickly raise blood glucose levels. However, because a typical serving of watermelon contains relatively few carbohydrates, its Glycemic Load is low. This means that despite its high GI, the impact of watermelon on blood sugar is limited by its low carbohydrate content. Conversely, foods with a high Glycemic Load, such as large portions of potatoes or white rice, can lead to significant increases in blood sugar levels, even if their GI is not exceptionally high.

Incorporating foods with low GI and low GL into your diet can be beneficial for managing blood sugar levels. Low-GI foods are absorbed more slowly, leading to a steady release of glucose into the bloodstream, which helps prevent the rapid fluctuations associated with high-GI foods. Additionally, low-GL foods reduce the overall carbohydrate load in a meal, further aiding in blood sugar control.

NOTE: Understanding both GI and GL allows for better dietary choices, particularly for individuals with diabetes or those looking to manage their weight and energy levels. By focusing on foods that have a low GI and GL, you can help maintain more stable blood sugar levels, improve overall health, and reduce the risk of developing chronic conditions related to blood sugar imbalances.

Hormones Involved In Blood Sugar Regulation

Hormones play a crucial role in regulating blood sugar levels, ensuring that our bodies maintain energy balance and metabolic stability. The primary hormone responsible for blood sugar regulation is insulin. Insulin is produced by the pancreas, an organ located near the stomach. When we consume food, particularly carbohydrates, these nutrients are broken down into glucose, which then enters the bloodstream. To manage this influx of glucose, the pancreas releases insulin. This hormone facilitates the uptake of glucose into cells, where it can be used for energy or stored for future use. By enabling cells to absorb glucose, insulin effectively lowers blood sugar levels, preventing hyperglycemia and maintaining a stable internal environment.

In contrast to insulin, another key hormone involved in blood sugar regulation is glucagon. Also produced by the pancreas, glucagon works to counteract the effects of insulin. When blood sugar levels fall, such as between meals or during periods of fasting, glucagon is secreted. It signals the liver to release stored glucose, known as glycogen, into the bloodstream. This release ensures a continuous supply of energy and helps to prevent hypoglycemia, thus maintaining equilibrium in blood sugar levels.

Beyond insulin and glucagon, other hormones also influence blood sugar regulation. Cortisol, commonly referred to as the "stress hormone," plays a role in elevating blood sugar levels. During stressful situations or times of increased demand, cortisol stimulates the liver to produce more glucose, which can contribute to higher blood sugar levels. This mechanism ensures that the body has enough energy to respond to stressors, but chronic stress can lead to persistent elevated blood sugar levels, which may contribute to health issues like diabetes.

Similarly, adrenaline, or epinephrine, is released during the "fight or flight" response. This hormone also increases blood sugar levels by promoting glucose production in the liver. Adrenaline's primary role is to prepare the body for immediate physical activity by providing a rapid energy source. Like cortisol, while adrenaline's effects are crucial for acute stress responses, excessive or prolonged exposure to high levels of adrenaline can adversely affect blood sugar control.

The Impact Of Carbohydrates On Blood Sugar

Carbohydrates are a primary source of energy for the body, but they can significantly affect blood sugar levels. Understanding their impact is crucial for maintaining balanced blood sugar and overall health. Carbohydrates come in two main forms: simple and complex.

Simple Carbohydrates

Simple carbohydrates are composed of one or two sugar units and are rapidly digested and absorbed by the body. Foods high in simple carbohydrates, such as candy, soda, and other sugary snacks, cause a swift increase in blood sugar levels. When consumed, these sugars are quickly broken down into glucose, resulting in a rapid spike in blood sugar. This swift increase is often followed by a rapid drop, which can lead to feelings of fatigue and hunger shortly after eating. Regular consumption of high-sugar foods can contribute to long-term issues such as insulin resistance and type 2 diabetes.

Complex Carbohydrates

Complex carbohydrates, on the other hand, consist of longer chains of sugar units. They are found in foods like whole grains, legumes, and vegetables. Because these carbohydrates are made up of more complex structures, they take longer for the body to break down and digest. As a result, glucose from complex carbohydrates is released more slowly into the bloodstream, leading to a gradual and more controlled increase in blood sugar levels. This slower digestion process helps maintain more stable blood sugar levels and can provide longer-lasting energy.

The Role of Fiber

Fiber, a type of carbohydrate that the body cannot digest, plays an essential role in blood sugar management. It is found in high amounts in vegetables, fruits, legumes, and whole grains. Fiber slows down the absorption of glucose in the digestive tract, which helps prevent sudden spikes in blood sugar levels. By including high-fiber foods in your diet, you can improve overall blood sugar control. Fiber also promotes digestive health, supports weight management, and contributes to heart health.

Balancing Carbohydrates for Better Health

To manage blood sugar effectively, it is important to balance the types and amounts of carbohydrates consumed. Favoring complex carbohydrates and high-fiber foods over simple sugars can lead to more stable blood sugar levels and better overall health. Incorporating a variety of nutrient-dense carbohydrates into your diet ensures you get essential vitamins, minerals, and energy while supporting blood sugar regulation.

The Role Of Proteins And Fats

Proteins and fats play crucial roles in managing blood sugar levels, even though carbohydrates have the most direct impact. While carbohydrates are the primary driver of blood sugar fluctuations, proteins and fats can significantly influence how the body processes glucose.

Proteins, which are abundant in foods like meat, dairy products, and legumes, generally have a minimal direct effect on blood sugar levels. However, their influence extends beyond this. When proteins are consumed alongside carbohydrates, they can affect the body's glycemic response. Proteins slow the digestion and absorption of carbohydrates, leading to a more gradual release of glucose into the bloodstream. This gradual increase helps prevent sharp spikes in blood sugar, which can be beneficial for managing conditions such as diabetes. By moderating glucose absorption, proteins contribute to a steadier and more controlled blood sugar level.

Fats, found in oils, butter, avocados, and nuts, also have a minimal direct impact on blood sugar levels. Their role in blood sugar management is somewhat similar to that of proteins. Fats slow the digestion process of carbohydrates, leading to a slower, more gradual rise in blood sugar. This slow digestion helps prevent rapid fluctuations in glucose levels, contributing to better blood sugar control.

Moreover, healthy fats, such as those present in nuts, seeds, and olive oil, offer additional benefits beyond their effects on blood sugar. These fats are essential for overall health and have been shown to improve insulin sensitivity. Insulin sensitivity is a critical factor in how effectively the body manages blood sugar. Improved insulin sensitivity means that the body's cells respond more efficiently to insulin, making it easier to regulate blood sugar levels.

Incorporating healthy fats into your diet can thus support overall metabolic health and contribute to better blood sugar management. For example, monounsaturated fats found in olive oil and avocados can enhance the body's ability to use insulin effectively, which is vital for maintaining balanced blood sugar levels.

CHAPTER THREE

ASSESSING YOUR BLOOD SUGAR

How To Monitor Your Blood Sugar Levels

Monitoring your blood sugar levels regularly is a crucial aspect of managing your health, especially if you have diabetes or other conditions that affect blood glucose levels. Keeping track of your blood sugar can help you understand how your diet, physical activity, and medications affect your glucose levels, thereby enabling you to make informed decisions about your health. One of the most common and effective methods for monitoring blood sugar is using a glucose meter. Here's a detailed guide to help you understand how to use a glucose meter effectively:

Step 1: Wash Your Hands

Before testing your blood sugar, it is essential to wash your hands thoroughly with soap and water. Clean hands prevent contamination and ensure that the blood sample is not affected by any substances on your skin, such as food residue or lotions, which could potentially alter the test results. After washing, dry your hands completely as wet fingers can dilute the blood sample, leading to inaccurate readings.

Step 2: Prepare the Glucose Meter

Next, prepare your glucose meter. Begin by inserting a test strip into the meter. Ensure that the meter is calibrated according to the manufacturer's instructions. Calibration is critical for the accuracy of the readings. Most modern glucose meters are user-friendly and come with detailed instructions for proper calibration. Some meters might require coding or using a control solution to verify that the device is working correctly.

Step 3: Prick Your Finger

Using a lancet, prick the side of your fingertip. This area tends to be less sensitive than the pad of your finger, making the process slightly less painful. Some glucose meters allow for alternative site testing, such as the forearm or the palm, which can be advantageous if you need to test frequently and want to avoid sore fingertips. Follow the specific instructions provided with your glucose meter for alternative site testing to ensure accurate results.

Step 4: Apply Blood to the Test Strip

After pricking your finger, gently squeeze it to obtain a small drop of blood. Carefully apply this drop to the test strip. Be sure to follow the meter's instructions regarding the amount of blood needed; too little can result in an error, and too much might cause the meter to malfunction. Most glucose meters are designed to require only a tiny drop of blood, making the process quick and minimally invasive.

Step 5: Read the Results

Within a few seconds, the glucose meter will display your blood sugar level. It is essential to record this number along with the date and time of the test. Keeping a log of your readings can help you and your healthcare provider track trends and make necessary adjustments to your treatment plan. Many people use a logbook or digital app to maintain their records. Digital apps often provide additional features such as graphs, reminders, and the ability to share data with healthcare professionals.

Understanding Blood Sugar Tests

Blood sugar tests are crucial for diagnosing and managing diabetes and other blood sugar-related conditions. There are several types of tests, each designed to provide specific insights into your blood sugar levels. Here's an overview of the main tests:

Fasting Blood Sugar Test

The fasting blood sugar test measures your blood sugar levels after an overnight fast, typically 8 to 12 hours without eating. It is one of the most common tests used to detect diabetes or prediabetes. The test is usually performed in the morning before breakfast. A normal fasting blood sugar level is below 100 mg/dL. Levels between 100 and 125 mg/dL are considered to indicate prediabetes, a condition where blood sugar levels are higher than normal but not yet high enough to be classified as diabetes. If your fasting blood sugar level is 126 mg/dL or higher on two separate tests, it is a strong indicator of diabetes. Regular monitoring through fasting blood sugar tests can help manage and adjust treatment plans effectively.

Postprandial Blood Sugar Test

The postprandial blood sugar test measures your blood sugar levels two hours after eating a meal. This test helps determine how your body responds to glucose intake from food. A normal postprandial blood sugar level is below 140 mg/dL. Levels between 140 and 199 mg/dL suggest prediabetes, indicating that your body is not processing glucose efficiently. Levels above 200 mg/dL are indicative of diabetes. This test is particularly useful in understanding the effectiveness of your current dietary choices and can help tailor meal plans to better control blood sugar levels.

A1C Test (Hemoglobin A1c)

The A1C test, also known as the hemoglobin A1c test, provides an average blood sugar level over the past two to three months. This test measures the percentage of hemoglobin in your blood that is coated with sugar (glycated). It is a key indicator of long-term blood sugar control and is often used to diagnose and monitor diabetes. A normal A1C level is below 5.7%. Levels between 5.7% and 6.4% indicate prediabetes, suggesting an increased risk of developing diabetes. An A1C level of 6.5% or higher on two separate tests suggests diabetes. The A1C test is particularly valuable as it does not require fasting and provides a broader picture of blood sugar management over time, unlike the daily fluctuations captured by fasting or postprandial tests.

Identifying Your Blood Sugar Triggers

Identifying what triggers changes in your blood sugar levels is crucial for effective management. Various factors can influence these levels, and understanding them can help you take control of your health.

Food and Drink: Carbohydrates significantly impact blood sugar levels. Foods such as bread, pasta, fruit, and sugary beverages can cause spikes. Carbohydrates are broken down into glucose, which enters the bloodstream, raising blood sugar levels. To manage this, monitor your carbohydrate intake carefully. Opt for complex carbohydrates found in whole grains and vegetables, as they are digested more slowly, leading to a gradual increase in blood sugar. Incorporating lean proteins and healthy fats can also help stabilize blood sugar levels. Pay attention to portion sizes and consider using a glycemic index chart to choose foods that have a lower impact on your blood sugar.

Physical Activity: Exercise generally lowers blood sugar levels by increasing insulin sensitivity, allowing cells to use available insulin more effectively. Regular physical activity, such as walking, swimming, or cycling, can help maintain stable blood sugar levels. However, intense or prolonged physical activity can sometimes temporarily raise blood sugar levels. This happens because the body releases stress hormones, like adrenaline, during intense exercise, which can prompt the liver to release glucose. Monitoring your blood sugar before, during, and after exercise can help you understand how different activities affect you and enable you to make necessary adjustments.

Stress: Stress can have a significant impact on blood sugar levels. When you are stressed, your body releases hormones like cortisol and adrenaline, which can cause an increase in blood sugar. This response is part of the body's "fight or flight" mechanism, which prepares you to deal with immediate threats. Chronic stress can lead to consistently elevated blood sugar levels, which can be harmful over time. Incorporating stress-reducing activities into your daily routine can help mitigate this effect. Practices such as meditation, yoga, deep breathing exercises, or even hobbies that you enjoy can reduce stress and help manage your blood sugar levels more effectively.

Illness: Being sick can also raise blood sugar levels. When your body is fighting an infection, it releases stress hormones, which can cause blood sugar to rise. This response is part of the immune system's effort to combat the illness. Additionally, factors like dehydration and reduced physical activity when you are unwell can contribute to higher blood sugar levels. It's essential to stay hydrated and follow your doctor's advice on managing blood sugar levels during illness. Regular monitoring is crucial, as you may need to adjust your medication or insulin dosage based on your readings.

Medications: Some medications can affect blood sugar levels. For instance, steroids and certain diuretics can cause an increase in blood sugar. If you are taking medications that may impact your blood sugar levels, it is vital to discuss potential side effects with your doctor. They can provide guidance on how to manage these effects and adjust your treatment plan if necessary. Always inform your healthcare provider about all the medications you are taking, including over-the-counter drugs and supplements, to ensure comprehensive management of your blood sugar levels.

Setting Realistic Goals For Blood Sugar Control

Managing blood sugar levels effectively involves setting realistic and achievable goals. This process is essential for maintaining overall health, especially for those with diabetes or other blood sugar-related conditions. Here are some comprehensive tips to help you set and achieve these goals successfully.

Consult with Your Doctor

The first step in setting realistic blood sugar goals is to consult with your healthcare provider. Your doctor can help you establish personalized blood sugar targets that consider your age, overall health status, lifestyle, and any existing medical conditions. Personalized goals are more achievable and effective because they are tailored to your unique needs. For instance, a target for an elderly person with multiple health issues might differ significantly from that for a younger, more active individual.

Set Specific Goals

When setting goals, specificity is key. Vague objectives such as "lower my blood sugar" can be difficult to measure and achieve. Instead, set clear, specific targets. For example, aim to maintain fasting blood sugar levels below 100 mg/dL or post-meal levels below 140 mg/dL. Specific goals provide a concrete target to work towards, making it easier to monitor progress and adjust your strategies as needed.

Track Your Progress

Keeping a detailed log of your blood sugar readings is crucial. Record not only your blood sugar levels but also your diet, exercise, medication, and other factors that might influence these levels. This comprehensive tracking helps you identify patterns and understand how different activities and foods impact your blood sugar. By analyzing this data, you can make informed adjustments to your lifestyle and treatment plan, enhancing your ability to maintain control over your blood sugar levels.

Make Gradual Changes

Implementing changes gradually is important to avoid feeling overwhelmed. Sudden, drastic changes can be difficult to sustain and may lead to frustration. Start with small, manageable adjustments. For example, begin by incorporating more vegetables into your meals or adding a 10-minute walk to your daily routine. Gradual changes are more likely to become permanent habits, leading to long-term improvements in blood sugar management.

Stay Positive and Motivated

Managing blood sugar levels is a long-term commitment that requires ongoing effort and motivation. Staying positive and celebrating small victories can help maintain your motivation. Focus on the positive changes in your health and well-being, such as increased energy levels or improved mood. These small successes can provide the encouragement needed to stay committed to your goals.

CHAPTER FOUR

DIETARY STRATEGIES FOR BLOOD SUGAR CONTROL

Low-Glycemic Foods And Their Benefits

Low-Glycemic Foods and Their Benefits

The glycemic index (GI) is a vital tool for understanding how different foods affect blood sugar levels. Foods are ranked on a scale from 0 to 100, with higher values indicating a more rapid increase in blood sugar. Low-GI foods, which have a slower and more gradual impact, can help maintain steady blood sugar levels and prevent spikes, offering numerous health benefits. These foods generally include whole grains, legumes, vegetables, and most fruits.

Whole Grains

Whole grains such as oatmeal, quinoa, and barley are excellent choices for those looking to manage their blood sugar levels. Unlike refined grains, whole grains retain their bran and germ, which contain valuable nutrients and fiber. This fiber content is key to their low GI rating, as it slows digestion and glucose absorption, providing a more sustained release of energy. Incorporating whole grains into your diet can help avoid the rapid increases in blood sugar that are often associated with refined grain products like white bread and rice.

Legumes

Legumes, including beans, lentils, and chickpeas, are another group of low-GI foods that are beneficial for blood sugar control. They are high in protein and fiber, two components that slow digestion and the absorption of glucose. This results in a more gradual increase in blood sugar levels post-meal. Moreover, legumes are rich in essential nutrients such as iron, magnesium, and potassium, which contribute to overall health. Regular consumption of legumes can also aid in weight management and reduce the risk of chronic diseases such as heart disease and diabetes.

Vegetables

Non-starchy vegetables are some of the best foods for maintaining low blood sugar levels. Vegetables like broccoli, spinach, and peppers are low in carbohydrates and high in fiber, making them ideal for blood sugar control. These vegetables have a minimal impact on blood sugar levels and are packed with essential vitamins and minerals, as well as antioxidants that support overall health. Consuming a variety of non-starchy vegetables daily can help enhance satiety, reduce calorie intake, and promote a healthy weight.

Fruits

While fruits contain natural sugars, many have a low GI and can be included in a blood sugar-friendly diet. Berries, apples, and pears, for example, are high in fiber and water, which helps moderate their impact on blood sugar levels. The key to consuming fruits as part of a low-GI diet is moderation and choosing fruits with a lower GI. These fruits provide important vitamins, minerals, and antioxidants that contribute to overall health. It's important to consume them in appropriate portions to manage sugar intake effectively.

Meal Planning And Portion Control

Meal planning and portion control are critical strategies for managing blood sugar levels, particularly for individuals with diabetes or those looking to maintain healthy blood glucose. By thoughtfully selecting and portioning meals, one can prevent overeating and ensure a balanced intake of essential nutrients.

Balanced Meals: Aiming for a balance of carbohydrates, proteins, and fats in each meal is essential. Proteins and fats slow the digestion of carbohydrates, resulting in a more gradual rise in blood sugar. A well-balanced meal might include a piece of grilled chicken (protein), a small serving of brown rice (carbohydrate), and a side of sautéed vegetables (fiber and vitamins). Including fiber-rich foods is also beneficial as fiber slows down the absorption of sugar, further stabilizing blood glucose levels. Leafy greens, whole grains, and legumes are excellent sources of fiber that can be easily incorporated into meals.

Regular Meals: Eating at regular intervals, typically every 3 to 4 hours, can help maintain stable blood sugar levels. Skipping meals can cause significant fluctuations in blood sugar, leading to both hyperglycemia and hypoglycemia. Consistency in meal timing helps the body manage insulin and blood sugar more effectively. For instance, having breakfast, a mid-morning snack, lunch, an afternoon snack, and dinner at consistent times each day can create a routine that the body responds to positively.

Portion Control: Using measuring cups or a food scale to ensure proper portion sizes is crucial. For example, one serving of cooked pasta is about half a cup. Being mindful of portion sizes can prevent excessive calorie intake, which is important for maintaining a healthy weight—a factor closely linked to blood sugar control. Visual cues can also help; for instance, a portion of protein should be about the size of a deck of cards, and a serving of vegetables can be as large as your fist. These guidelines help keep portions in check without the need for constant measuring.

Healthy Snacks: Choosing snacks that combine protein and fiber can help prevent blood sugar spikes and keep you feeling full between meals. For example, a small handful of nuts with an apple is a great option. The fiber in the apple and the protein and healthy fats in the nuts work together to slow down the absorption of sugar, providing sustained energy and satiety. Other healthy snack options include Greek yogurt with berries, hummus with carrot sticks, or a small serving of cottage cheese with cucumber slices.

The Importance Of Fiber

Fiber is a crucial component in the management of blood sugar levels. It operates by slowing the absorption of sugar into the bloodstream, thereby preventing rapid spikes in blood glucose. Understanding the different types of fiber and their respective benefits is essential for anyone looking to maintain stable blood sugar levels and overall health.

Fiber is categorized into two main types: soluble and insoluble. Each type plays a unique role in the body. Soluble fiber dissolves in water to form a gel-like substance. This gel can help lower blood sugar levels by slowing down the absorption of sugar. Additionally, soluble fiber is known to reduce cholesterol levels, contributing to cardiovascular health. Excellent sources of soluble fiber include oats, barley, beans, lentils, apples, and citrus fruits. These foods not only provide fiber but also come packed with various vitamins and minerals, making them a valuable addition to a balanced diet.

On the other hand, insoluble fiber does not dissolve in water. Instead, it adds bulk to the stool and aids in regular bowel movements. This type of fiber helps prevent constipation and supports a healthy digestive system. Foods rich in insoluble fiber include whole grains, nuts, and vegetables like carrots and broccoli. These foods help maintain a healthy digestive tract and can prevent gastrointestinal issues such as diverticulosis and hemorrhoids.

Incorporating an adequate amount of fiber into your diet is essential for reaping these health benefits. The recommended daily intake of fiber is at least 25-30 grams. This can be achieved by including a variety of fiber-rich foods in your daily meals. For instance, starting your day with a bowl of oatmeal topped with fruits can provide a significant amount of soluble fiber.

Snacking on a handful of nuts or a piece of fruit like an apple or orange can further boost your fiber intake. Including vegetables in every meal, opting for whole grains over refined grains, and adding legumes like beans and lentils to soups and salads are effective ways to meet your daily fiber requirements.

Fiber also plays a role in weight management. High-fiber foods are generally more filling than low-fiber foods, which can help control appetite and reduce overall calorie intake. This is particularly beneficial for those looking to lose weight or maintain a healthy weight. Additionally, a diet high in fiber has been associated with a reduced risk of developing chronic diseases such as type 2 diabetes, heart disease, and certain types of cancer.

Superfoods For Blood Sugar Management

Managing blood sugar levels is crucial for overall health, particularly for those with diabetes or insulin resistance. Incorporating superfoods into your diet can offer additional support in regulating glucose levels. Here's a closer look at some of these beneficial superfoods and how they can enhance your blood sugar management.

Cinnamon is renowned for its potential to improve insulin sensitivity and lower blood sugar levels. Research indicates that the compounds in cinnamon may mimic insulin's effects and increase glucose uptake by cells. Incorporating cinnamon into your daily diet is easy and delicious. Sprinkle it on your morning oatmeal, blend it into smoothies, or use it in your baking to add a sweet, aromatic flavor while benefiting your blood sugar control.

Chia Seeds are a nutritional powerhouse packed with fiber, omega-3 fatty acids, and essential nutrients. The high fiber content in chia seeds helps slow down the digestion and absorption of carbohydrates, leading to more stable blood sugar levels. They also offer a satisfying texture and can be easily incorporated into various dishes. Mix chia seeds into yogurt for a nutritious snack, blend them into your smoothies, or use them in baking to boost the fiber content of your recipes.

Turmeric contains curcumin, a compound with powerful anti-inflammatory and blood sugar-lowering properties. Curcumin may help improve insulin sensitivity and reduce inflammation, which is beneficial for managing blood sugar levels. You can include turmeric in your diet by adding it to curries, soups, and stews or by taking it as a supplement. Its vibrant yellow color and warm, earthy flavor make it a versatile ingredient in many dishes.

Leafy Greens, such as spinach, kale, and Swiss chard, are excellent choices for managing blood sugar. These vegetables are low in carbohydrates and high in fiber and essential nutrients. Their fiber content helps slow the absorption of sugar into the bloodstream, which can aid in stabilizing blood glucose levels. Incorporate leafy greens into your diet by adding them to salads, blending them into smoothies, or using them in stir-fries and soups.

Nuts like almonds and walnuts provide a combination of healthy fats, fiber, and protein, all of which contribute to stable blood sugar levels. The healthy fats in nuts help improve insulin sensitivity, while their fiber content slows the digestion of carbohydrates. Enjoy a small handful of nuts as a snack, or sprinkle them on salads and yogurt for an extra crunch and nutritional boost.

CHAPTER FIVE

CREATING BALANCED MEALS

Designing Breakfast For Stable Blood Sugar

Breakfast is often hailed as the most crucial meal of the day, and for good reason. It sets the stage for your energy levels and blood sugar balance throughout the day. To craft a breakfast that supports stable blood sugar, it's essential to focus on a balanced combination of protein, healthy fats, and complex carbohydrates.

Protein is a key component in stabilizing blood sugar. It works by slowing down the absorption of carbohydrates, which helps prevent sudden spikes and drops in blood sugar levels. High-protein options such as eggs, Greek yogurt, or tofu are excellent choices. For instance, a scrambled egg mixed with vegetables provides not only protein but also essential vitamins and minerals. Greek yogurt paired with fresh berries offers a tasty and satisfying start to your day while delivering a significant protein boost.

Healthy Fats are another crucial element. They help keep you full longer and provide a steady release of energy. Avocados, nuts, and seeds are great sources of healthy fats. Incorporating these into your breakfast can be simple yet effective. For example, a slice of whole-grain toast topped with mashed avocado creates a satisfying and nutrient-rich meal. Alternatively, a handful of almonds can be a convenient addition, enhancing the nutritional profile of your breakfast while helping to maintain blood sugar stability.

When it comes to Complex Carbohydrates, opting for whole grains and fruits is key. Unlike refined sugars, complex carbohydrates are digested more slowly, which helps to prevent sharp fluctuations in blood sugar levels. Good options include oatmeal, whole-grain cereals, or a piece of fruit paired with nut butter. Oatmeal provides sustained energy and fiber, which supports digestive health. A whole-grain cereal combined with milk or yogurt offers a balanced mix of nutrients. A piece of fruit, such as an apple or banana, with a dollop of almond butter can satisfy your sweet tooth while delivering both fiber and protein.

Lunch Options To Prevent Afternoon Slumps

Lunch plays a crucial role in maintaining energy levels and avoiding that dreaded afternoon slump. To keep your blood sugar stable and prevent feeling sluggish, it's essential to focus on a balanced mix of protein, fiber, and healthy fats. Here's how you can craft a lunch that supports sustained energy throughout the day:

Protein: Lean proteins are key to sustaining energy and supporting muscle function. Incorporate options such as chicken, turkey, fish, or plant-based alternatives like legumes and tofu into your lunch. These proteins help keep you full and energized. For instance, a grilled chicken salad provides not only protein but also essential vitamins and minerals from the fresh vegetables. Alternatively, a chickpea and quinoa bowl combines plant-based protein with whole grains, offering a nutritious and satisfying meal.

Fiber: Fiber is vital for regulating blood sugar levels by slowing down the digestion process. This helps prevent sudden spikes and crashes in your energy levels. To boost your fiber intake, incorporate fiber-rich vegetables, whole grains, and legumes into your lunch. A whole-grain wrap filled with an assortment of vegetables and beans offers a delicious and fiber-rich option. Another great choice is a hearty vegetable soup loaded with beans. This type of meal not only provides fiber but also keeps you full longer, aiding in the prevention of the afternoon slump.

Healthy Fats: Including healthy fats in your lunch can enhance the flavor and keep you satisfied for longer. Sources of healthy fats like olive oil, avocados, or nuts are beneficial additions to your meal. A drizzle of olive oil on your salad not only adds a tasty element but also provides healthy fats that help maintain energy levels. Similarly, adding a small handful of walnuts to your soup or salad can provide a satisfying crunch and a boost of healthy fats.

Dinner Ideas For Sustained Energy

When planning dinner to ensure sustained energy throughout the evening, it's important to focus on a balanced meal that includes protein, complex carbohydrates, and a variety of vegetables. This combination not only supports energy levels but also aids in recovery and overall well-being.

Protein: The foundation of a sustaining dinner should be lean proteins. Opt for choices such as fish, poultry, or plant-based proteins. For instance, baked salmon is an excellent option, rich in omega-3 fatty acids, which are beneficial for heart health and can help improve mood and cognitive function. Alternatively, a hearty lentil stew can be a nutritious plant-based option. Lentils are high in protein and fiber, which contribute to satiety and steady energy release. If you prefer poultry, grilled chicken breast or turkey can provide the necessary protein without excess fat.

Complex Carbohydrates: Including complex carbohydrates in your dinner is crucial for maintaining energy levels. Unlike simple carbohydrates, complex carbs are digested more slowly, providing a steady release of glucose into the bloodstream. Brown rice is a great choice, offering not only energy but also essential nutrients like B vitamins and magnesium. Sweet potatoes are another excellent option; they are rich in beta-carotene, fiber, and antioxidants. Whole-grain pasta is also beneficial, as it provides sustained energy and supports digestive health. A side of roasted sweet potatoes or a serving of quinoa can complement your main dish, ensuring you have a well-rounded meal.

Vegetables: To complete your dinner, incorporate a variety of vegetables. Vegetables are packed with essential vitamins, minerals, and fiber, all of which play a role in maintaining overall health and supporting energy levels. Steamed broccoli, for instance, is rich in vitamins C and K, as well as fiber, which aids in digestion and helps keep you full. Sautéed spinach is another excellent choice; it contains iron and folate, important for energy production and reducing fatigue. For a more colorful and diverse option, consider a mixed vegetable stir-fry. This can include bell peppers, carrots, and snap peas, adding not only nutritional value but also a variety of textures and flavors to your meal.

Healthy Snacks To Keep Blood Sugar In Check

Maintaining steady blood sugar levels throughout the day is crucial for overall health and well-being. Healthy snacks play an important role in this, helping to bridge the gap between meals and prevent blood sugar dips. The key to effective snacking lies in choosing options that offer a balanced combination of protein, healthy fats, and fiber.

Protein-Rich Snacks

Incorporating protein into your snacks can be a game-changer for blood sugar control. Protein helps stabilize blood sugar levels by slowing down the absorption of glucose into the bloodstream. Simple yet effective options include a handful of nuts, a piece of cheese, or a boiled egg. Nuts like almonds, walnuts, and pistachios are not only rich in protein but also provide essential vitamins and minerals. A piece of cheese, such as string cheese or a slice of cheddar, offers a satisfying and protein-packed choice. For a quick, portable snack, a boiled egg delivers high-quality protein and is easy to prepare in advance.

Healthy Fats

Adding sources of healthy fats to your snacks can enhance satisfaction and support stable blood sugar levels. Healthy fats contribute to satiety and can help manage hunger between meals. Nut butters, seeds, and avocados are excellent choices. For instance, pairing a small apple with almond butter creates a satisfying snack that combines the natural sweetness of the apple with the creamy richness of the nut butter. Similarly, spreading a few slices of avocado on whole-grain crackers provides a delicious and nutritious option. These fats also offer essential fatty acids that are beneficial for overall health.

Fiber-Rich Choices

Fiber is another crucial component for managing blood sugar levels. It helps slow down the digestion and absorption of carbohydrates, leading to more stable blood sugar levels. Snacks that are high in fiber include raw vegetables, fruits, and whole-grain options. Carrot sticks paired with hummus make for a crunchy, fiber-rich snack that also provides protein from the hummus. Alternatively, enjoying a piece of fruit along with a small handful of nuts combines fiber with protein and healthy fats, creating a well-rounded snack. Whole-grain snacks, such as whole-grain crackers or popcorn, are also great options that offer sustained energy and fiber.

CHAPTER SIX

EXERCISE AND BLOOD SUGAR

The Benefits Of Physical Activity

Physical activity offers numerous benefits for managing blood sugar levels, with its impact on insulin sensitivity being one of the most notable advantages. Insulin, a crucial hormone produced by the pancreas, helps cells absorb glucose from the bloodstream. When physical activity is incorporated into daily routines, muscles become more responsive to insulin. This increased sensitivity allows cells to take up glucose more effectively, which in turn helps to lower blood sugar levels. As a result, regular exercise plays a significant role in regulating blood glucose and preventing spikes.

Another key benefit of physical activity is its effectiveness in weight management. Excess body weight, particularly around the abdomen, is a major risk factor for the development of type 2 diabetes. Engaging in regular exercise aids in maintaining a healthy weight by burning calories and improving the body's metabolism. By reducing body fat and supporting lean muscle growth, physical activity can help manage and lower the risk of developing diabetes. This contributes to overall metabolic health, enhancing the body's ability to regulate blood sugar.

In addition to improving insulin sensitivity and aiding in weight control, exercise plays a critical role in stress management. Stress can adversely affect blood sugar levels by triggering the release of stress hormones, such as cortisol. Elevated cortisol levels can lead to increased blood glucose levels, making it challenging to maintain stable blood sugar. Physical activity serves as a natural stress reliever, helping to reduce the levels of these stress hormones. By incorporating exercise into your routine, you can mitigate the negative effects of stress on blood sugar, contributing to a more balanced and stable glucose level.

Types Of Exercise For Blood Sugar Control

Incorporating a variety of exercise types into your routine can play a crucial role in managing blood sugar levels and overall health. Three primary categories— aerobic, resistance, and flexibility exercises—each contribute uniquely to blood sugar control and metabolic health.

Aerobic Exercise: Aerobic activities, such as walking, jogging, cycling, and swimming, are highly effective for improving cardiovascular health and managing blood sugar levels. These exercises increase your heart rate and enhance circulation, which helps muscles utilize glucose more efficiently. Aerobic exercise stimulates insulin production and promotes better glucose uptake by cells. For optimal benefits, aim to engage in at least 150 minutes of moderate-intensity aerobic exercise per week. This duration can be broken down into manageable sessions, such as 30 minutes a day, five days a week. Regular aerobic activity not only supports blood sugar control but also boosts overall energy levels and mood.

Resistance Training: Strength training exercises, including weight lifting and bodyweight exercises, are essential for building muscle mass. Increased muscle mass improves the body's ability to store and use glucose, leading to better blood sugar regulation. Muscle cells are more sensitive to insulin, which helps in effective glucose uptake and storage. Incorporating resistance training into your routine 2-3 times a week can significantly enhance insulin sensitivity and support long-term blood sugar management. This type of exercise also contributes to increased metabolism, improved muscle tone, and overall physical strength.

Flexibility and Balance Exercises: Flexibility and balance exercises, such as yoga and stretching, may not have a direct impact on blood sugar levels but are valuable for overall health. These activities improve flexibility, balance, and coordination, which can reduce the risk of injury and enhance physical function. While they might not directly affect glucose metabolism, they complement aerobic and resistance exercises by supporting overall well-being and recovery. Regular practice of yoga or stretching can also reduce stress, which is beneficial for blood sugar control as stress can negatively impact glucose levels.

Creating An Exercise Routine

Developing a consistent exercise routine is crucial for effectively managing blood sugar levels. To begin, it's essential to set realistic and achievable goals. Start with manageable objectives and gradually increase the intensity and duration of your workouts as your fitness improves. This progressive approach helps in building endurance while reducing the risk of injury or burnout.

Choosing activities you genuinely enjoy is key to maintaining motivation and consistency. Whether it's walking, cycling, swimming, or a fitness class, engaging in enjoyable exercises will make it easier to stick to your routine. Incorporating a variety of activities can also prevent boredom and keep your routine fresh and exciting.

Timing is another important factor to consider when planning your exercise sessions. For optimal blood sugar management, schedule your workouts at times when your blood sugar levels are typically stable. This might mean exercising before meals for some individuals, while others may find it more beneficial to work out after eating. It's important to monitor how your blood sugar responds to different types of exercise and their timing. This personalized approach allows you to adjust your routine to achieve the best results for your specific needs.

Hydration and nutrition play significant roles in supporting your exercise routine and overall health. Staying well-hydrated helps your body perform optimally during physical activity and aids in recovery afterward. Additionally, consuming a balanced meal or snack before and after exercising helps regulate blood sugar levels and provides the necessary energy for your workouts. Opt for foods that combine carbohydrates with protein and healthy fats to sustain energy levels and support muscle recovery.

Moreover, incorporating regular exercise into your daily routine can contribute to improved insulin sensitivity and better blood sugar control. Aim for at least 150 minutes of moderate-intensity aerobic activity per week, along with muscle-strengthening exercises on two or more days. These recommendations align with guidelines from health organizations and are supported by research on effective blood sugar management through physical activity.

Monitoring Blood Sugar During Exercise

Monitoring blood sugar levels during exercise is especially important for individuals with diabetes, as physical activity can significantly impact glucose levels. Understanding how exercise affects your blood sugar and implementing proper monitoring strategies can help maintain stability and avoid complications.

Pre-Exercise Blood Sugar Check

Before beginning any exercise routine, it's crucial to check your blood sugar levels. Aim to ensure that your glucose is within a safe range to avoid potential issues. If your blood sugar is too low, known as hypoglycemia, consider having a small snack or carbohydrate-rich food to bring it up to a safer level. This precaution helps prevent low blood sugar during your workout, which can lead to dizziness, weakness, or even fainting.

Conversely, if your blood sugar levels are too high, known as hyperglycemia, it might be wise to delay your exercise until they stabilize. High glucose levels can be dangerous and may increase the risk of complications during physical activity. In such cases, focus on managing your blood sugar through appropriate medication, hydration, and perhaps a light walk rather than high-intensity exercise.

During Exercise: Regular Monitoring

While exercising, especially if engaging in high-intensity activities or prolonged sessions, it's advisable to periodically check your blood sugar levels. Physical activity can cause fluctuations in glucose levels, which can sometimes be unpredictable. Regular monitoring helps in promptly addressing any sudden changes and adjusting your activity level or intake as needed.

If you notice symptoms of hypoglycemia, such as dizziness, shaking, excessive sweating, or confusion, it's crucial to stop exercising and check your blood sugar immediately. Consuming a quick source of carbohydrates, such as a glucose tablet or a sugary drink, can help raise your blood sugar levels quickly.

Post-Exercise Blood Sugar Monitoring

After completing your exercise, it's important to check your blood sugar levels again. Exercise can have lingering effects on glucose levels, and monitoring ensures that your blood sugar remains within a safe range post-workout. Depending on the intensity and duration of the exercise, your blood sugar may continue to fluctuate, so keeping track helps in making any necessary adjustments to your post-exercise nutrition or medication.

CHAPTER SEVEN

MANAGING STRESS AND SLEEP

The Connection Between Stress And Blood Sugar

Stress has a profound impact on blood sugar levels, an issue of particular concern for individuals managing diabetes or other blood sugar-related conditions. The relationship between stress and blood sugar is primarily mediated through the release of stress hormones such as cortisol and adrenaline. These hormones are integral to the body's "fight or flight" response, designed to prepare us for immediate physical threats. However, in contemporary life, stress often arises from non-threatening sources such as work pressures, financial difficulties, or interpersonal conflicts. This chronic stress can continually trigger the release of these hormones, leading to sustained physiological responses.

Cortisol, one of the key stress hormones, plays a significant role in increasing blood sugar levels. When the body perceives a stressor, cortisol is released from the adrenal glands and signals the liver to produce more glucose. This increase in glucose is intended to provide a quick energy boost needed to deal with immediate threats. In the context of acute stress, this mechanism is beneficial, but when stress becomes chronic, it results in prolonged periods of elevated blood sugar levels. This is problematic for individuals with diabetes or those who are already at risk of developing blood sugar management issues.

In addition to the hormonal effects, stress often leads to unhealthy eating habits, which can exacerbate the problem. For instance, people under stress may gravitate toward sugary or high-carbohydrate foods as a form of comfort or due to a lack of time to prepare balanced meals. These dietary choices can lead to additional spikes in blood sugar levels, compounding the impact of stress on glycemic control.

Furthermore, the interplay between stress and blood sugar management can create a vicious cycle. Elevated blood sugar levels caused by stress can lead to feelings of fatigue and irritability, which can, in turn, increase stress levels further. This ongoing cycle can make it challenging for individuals to manage their blood sugar effectively and can contribute to the development or worsening of diabetes-related complications.

Techniques For Stress Reduction

Reducing stress is crucial for maintaining balanced blood sugar levels and overall well-being. Fortunately, several effective techniques can help manage stress and improve your quality of life.

Exercise is a powerful stress reliever. Engaging in physical activity triggers the release of endorphins, the body's natural mood enhancers. Regular exercise also lowers cortisol levels, a hormone associated with stress, and enhances insulin sensitivity, which is beneficial for blood sugar management. Aim for at least 30 minutes of moderate exercise most days of the week to harness these benefits.

Mindfulness and meditation are valuable tools for calming the mind and reducing stress. Mindfulness practices, including meditation, help in managing stress by focusing attention on the present moment and fostering emotional resilience. Techniques such as deep breathing, progressive muscle relaxation, and guided imagery can be particularly effective. These methods help in calming the nervous system and reducing the physiological impact of stress.

Healthy eating plays a significant role in stress management. A balanced diet rich in fruits, vegetables, whole grains, and lean proteins supports the body's stress response and overall health. Nutrient-dense foods provide the essential vitamins and minerals needed for a well-functioning stress response system. Conversely, excessive consumption of caffeine and sugar can exacerbate stress and lead to blood sugar imbalances. Maintaining a nutritious diet can thus help mitigate these effects and support better stress management.

Adequate sleep is another critical component of stress reduction. Quality sleep is essential for regulating stress hormones and maintaining a stable mood. Sleep deprivation can elevate cortisol levels, leading to increased stress and negative mood changes. Establishing a regular sleep routine and creating a calming bedtime environment can significantly enhance sleep quality, which in turn helps in managing stress more effectively.

Social support is invaluable for coping with stress. Engaging with friends, family, or a therapist provides emotional support and practical assistance. A strong social network offers comfort and helps in navigating stressors more effectively, fostering a sense of connection and support.

Hobbies and relaxation also play a vital role in stress management. Participating in activities that you enjoy, such as reading, gardening, or crafting, can provide a break from daily stressors and improve your mood. Making time for these enjoyable activities helps in diverting attention away from stress and contributes to overall well-being.

The Importance Of Sleep For Blood Sugar Control

Sleep is crucial for maintaining optimal blood sugar control. Insufficient or poor-quality sleep can significantly impact how effectively your body regulates blood sugar levels. During sleep, the body engages in vital processes that help balance hormones, including those that manage blood sugar.

When you don't get enough sleep, it disrupts the balance of hormones such as cortisol and insulin. Cortisol, often referred to as the "stress hormone," can increase when you are sleep-deprived. Elevated cortisol levels can lead to insulin resistance, making it more challenging for your body to manage blood sugar. This resistance impairs the body's ability to use insulin effectively, resulting in higher blood sugar levels.

Additionally, poor sleep affects hormones that regulate appetite, including ghrelin and leptin. Ghrelin stimulates hunger, while leptin signals satiety. Lack of sleep can cause an imbalance in these hormones, leading to increased hunger and cravings for high-carbohydrate and high-sugar foods. This can create a cycle of poor dietary choices that further disrupt blood sugar levels, exacerbating the issue.

Inadequate sleep also affects the body's ability to repair itself and maintain metabolic processes. During sleep, the body performs critical functions such as muscle repair, immune system strengthening, and hormone regulation. Disrupted sleep prevents these processes from occurring optimally, further impacting overall health and blood sugar control.

To support healthy blood sugar levels, it's essential to prioritize good sleep hygiene. Aim for 7-9 hours of uninterrupted sleep each night. Establishing a consistent sleep schedule, going to bed, and waking up at the same time every day can help regulate your internal body clock. Creating a relaxing bedtime routine, such as reading or taking a warm bath, can also improve sleep quality.

Creating A Sleep-Friendly Environment

Creating a sleep-friendly environment is crucial for achieving restful and rejuvenating sleep. By carefully designing your sleeping space and establishing a calming pre-sleep routine, you can significantly enhance your overall sleep quality. Here are several key strategies to help you create an ideal environment for rest:

1. Comfortable Bedding: Your choice of bedding plays a fundamental role in ensuring a good night's sleep. Invest in a high-quality mattress and pillows that offer adequate support and comfort. The right mattress should align with your body's natural curves and provide sufficient support to prevent discomfort and pain. Pillows should support your neck and head in a neutral position. Additionally, keep your bedding clean and fresh, as a tidy bed can be more inviting and relaxing.

2. Optimal Temperature: The temperature of your bedroom can greatly impact your sleep. Most people sleep best in a cool

environment, with the ideal temperature ranging between 60-67°F (15-19°C). To maintain this temperature, consider using a fan or air conditioning during warmer months, and a heater or extra blankets during colder months. Adjusting the room temperature to your comfort level can help you fall asleep faster and enjoy deeper sleep.

3. Darkness and Quiet: Creating a dark and quiet sleeping environment is essential for uninterrupted rest. Darkness helps regulate your body's internal clock, signaling that it's time to sleep. Use blackout curtains or an eye mask to block out any external light sources that might disrupt your sleep. Additionally, reduce noise disturbances by using earplugs or a white noise machine. These tools can help

mask background sounds that might otherwise wake you during the night.

4. Relaxing Routine: Establishing a soothing bedtime routine can signal to your body that it's time to wind down. Engaging in calming activities such as reading a book, taking a warm bath, or practicing relaxation techniques like deep breathing or meditation can help prepare your mind and body for sleep. Consistently following a pre-sleep routine can condition your body to recognize when it's time to transition from wakefulness to rest.

5. Limit Screen Time: The use of electronic devices before bed can interfere with your sleep-wake cycle due to the blue light emitted by screens. This light can suppress the production of melatonin, a hormone that regulates sleep. To mitigate this effect,

avoid using screens at least an hour before bedtime. Instead, opt for relaxing activities that don't involve screens to help your body prepare for restful sleep.

☐

CHAPTER EIGHT

SUPPLEMENTS AND NATURAL REMEDIES

Vitamins And Minerals For Blood Sugar Regulation

Maintaining healthy blood sugar levels is crucial for overall well-being, and vitamins and minerals play a significant role in this process. Several key nutrients are essential for optimal blood sugar regulation:

Chromium is a vital mineral that enhances insulin sensitivity and helps regulate blood sugar levels. Insulin is a hormone that allows cells to absorb glucose from the bloodstream. Chromium works by improving the efficiency of insulin, which helps to stabilize blood sugar levels. It is found in various foods, such as broccoli, whole grains, and meats. Additionally, chromium supplements are available for those who may not get enough from their diet.

Magnesium is another crucial mineral involved in glucose metabolism and insulin action. This mineral helps regulate how insulin interacts with cells, facilitating the uptake of glucose and ensuring proper energy production. A deficiency in magnesium can impair insulin sensitivity, leading to higher blood sugar levels and an increased risk of type 2 diabetes. Magnesium-rich foods include nuts, seeds, and leafy green vegetables, which can support healthy blood sugar levels.

Vitamin D is essential for insulin function and overall metabolic health. Research suggests that insufficient levels of vitamin D are linked to insulin resistance and type

2 diabetes. Vitamin D helps regulate the body's insulin production and function. Adequate levels of this vitamin can be maintained through moderate sun exposure and by consuming foods rich in vitamin D, such as fatty fish and fortified dairy products. Supplements can also be beneficial for those who struggle to obtain enough vitamin D from dietary sources or sunlight.

Alpha-Lipoic Acid (ALA) is a powerful antioxidant that plays a role in reducing oxidative stress and improving insulin sensitivity. Oxidative stress can damage cells and impair insulin action, contributing to high blood sugar levels. ALA helps mitigate these effects and supports better glucose control. It is found in foods such as spinach, broccoli, and red meat, and is also available as a supplement.

Herbal Supplements For Blood Sugar Control

Managing blood sugar levels is crucial for individuals with diabetes or those seeking to maintain metabolic health. While conventional treatments are often effective, several herbal supplements have shown promise in supporting blood sugar control. Here's a look at some of these supplements:

Cinnamon: Cinnamon is more than just a flavorful spice. Research suggests that cinnamon may play a role in improving insulin sensitivity, which can help regulate blood sugar levels. It is believed that compounds in cinnamon enhance the body's ability to utilize glucose efficiently.

To incorporate cinnamon into your routine, you can sprinkle it on foods or beverages, or take it in supplement form. It's worth noting that the type of cinnamon used, specifically Ceylon cinnamon, is preferred over Cassia cinnamon for its potential health benefits and lower coumarin content.

Berberine: Berberine is a bioactive compound found in several plants, including Goldenseal and Barberry. It has gained attention for its ability to enhance insulin sensitivity and regulate glucose metabolism. Studies have shown that berberine can be as effective as some pharmaceutical medications in lowering blood sugar levels. Berberine supplements are typically available in capsule or tablet form. Due to its strong biological activity, it's essential to follow dosage guidelines and consult with a healthcare provider before starting berberine.

Fenugreek: Fenugreek, a common herb used in cooking, is notable for its soluble fiber content, which may help manage blood sugar levels. The fiber in fenugreek seeds can slow down carbohydrate absorption, which helps improve insulin sensitivity and reduce post-meal blood sugar spikes. Fenugreek can be added to dishes as a spice or consumed as a supplement. It's also used in traditional medicine for its potential to support metabolic health and overall wellness.

Ginseng: Ginseng has been utilized in traditional medicine for centuries to support various aspects of health, including blood sugar control. Both

American ginseng and Asian ginseng are believed to improve glucose metabolism and enhance insulin sensitivity. Research indicates that ginseng may help lower fasting blood sugar levels and improve overall metabolic function. Ginseng supplements are available in various forms, including capsules, teas, and extracts. Choosing the right type of ginseng and proper dosage is crucial, so it's advisable to consult with a healthcare provider.

The Role Of Probiotics

Probiotics, often recognized for their role in supporting digestive health, are gaining attention for their potential impact on blood sugar regulation. These beneficial bacteria are integral to maintaining a balanced gut microbiome, which in turn can significantly influence glucose metabolism and insulin sensitivity.

A healthy gut microbiome is essential for optimal digestion and nutrient absorption. Probiotics contribute to this balance by supporting the growth of beneficial bacteria while inhibiting the growth of harmful microorganisms. This balance is crucial because it affects how effectively the body processes carbohydrates and absorbs nutrients, both of which can impact blood sugar levels. For example, a well-functioning gut can help ensure that nutrients are properly absorbed, which may prevent spikes in blood sugar levels following meals.

Moreover, probiotics may help reduce systemic inflammation, a condition commonly associated with insulin resistance and type 2 diabetes. Chronic inflammation can impair the body's ability to respond to insulin, a hormone responsible for regulating blood sugar levels. By promoting a healthier gut environment, probiotics may reduce inflammation and, consequently, improve insulin sensitivity. Research indicates that certain probiotic strains possess anti-inflammatory properties that can help mitigate systemic inflammation, thereby supporting better glucose control.

In addition to reducing inflammation, probiotics may enhance insulin sensitivity. Insulin sensitivity refers to how effectively the body responds to insulin. Some studies have shown that specific strains of probiotics can positively affect glucose metabolism, leading to improved insulin sensitivity. This is particularly important for individuals at risk of or managing type 2 diabetes, as improved insulin sensitivity can help maintain more stable blood sugar levels and reduce the risk of diabetes-related complications.

Using Natural Remedies Safely

Natural remedies, while often appealing for their holistic approach, require careful use to maximize their benefits and avoid potential risks. Here's a comprehensive guide on how to use natural remedies safely and effectively:

1. Consult a Healthcare Professional: Before incorporating any new supplement or herbal remedy into your routine, it is crucial to seek advice from a healthcare provider. This step is particularly important if you have existing health

conditions, are pregnant, or are taking prescription medications. A healthcare professional can provide personalized guidance, help you understand possible interactions with current treatments, and assess whether the natural remedy is suitable for your specific needs. This precaution ensures that you make informed decisions and avoid adverse effects.

2. Follow Dosage Recommendations: Adhering to recommended dosages is essential to ensure the safe use of natural remedies. Overuse or incorrect dosing can lead to unwanted side effects or interactions with other treatments. Dosage guidelines are typically based on clinical research or traditional usage, so it's important to follow these

recommendations carefully. If you are unsure about the appropriate dosage, consult your healthcare provider for clarification. Proper dosing helps you achieve the desired therapeutic effects while minimizing risks.

3. Monitor Blood Sugar Levels: If you are using natural remedies to manage conditions like diabetes, regular monitoring of your blood sugar levels is vital. This practice helps you determine if the supplements or remedies are having the intended effect and if they are causing any unexpected changes in your blood sugar. Consistent monitoring allows you to make adjustments as needed and ensures that your natural remedies are supporting your health without causing imbalances or other issues.

4. Choose Quality Products: The quality of the supplements you use can significantly impact their effectiveness and safety. Opt for products from reputable brands that prioritize quality control and transparency. Look for supplements that have undergone third-party testing to verify their purity and potency. This step helps you avoid products that may be contaminated or inaccurately labeled. Choosing high-quality supplements ensures that you are using remedies that are safe and effective.

CHAPTER NINE

SPECIAL CONSIDERATIONS

Managing Blood Sugar In Diabetes

Managing blood sugar is crucial for individuals with diabetes to maintain overall health and prevent complications. Effective blood sugar management involves a combination of dietary adjustments, physical activity, and medication. Regular monitoring of blood glucose levels is essential for tailoring these strategies to individual needs.

A well-balanced diet plays a pivotal role in regulating blood sugar levels. Foods rich in fiber, such as whole grains, vegetables, and legumes, are beneficial because they help stabilize glucose levels. Fiber slows down the absorption of sugars, leading to a more gradual rise in blood sugar. Reducing the intake of refined sugars and processed foods is also important. These foods can cause rapid spikes in blood glucose levels, making it harder to manage diabetes. Carbohydrate counting is a common technique where individuals track the amount of carbohydrates they consume. This practice helps in making informed dietary choices and managing blood sugar more effectively.

Physical activity is another critical component in blood sugar management. Regular exercise enhances insulin sensitivity, which means the body can use blood sugar more efficiently. A combination of aerobic exercises, like walking or cycling, and strength training is recommended. Aerobic exercises help with cardiovascular health and weight management, while strength training builds muscle, which can further improve insulin sensitivity. Monitoring blood sugar levels before and after exercise is important, as physical activity can lead to fluctuations in blood glucose.

Medication management is integral to controlling diabetes. Individuals may need to take oral medications or insulin injections based on their specific type of diabetes and treatment plan. Adhering to the prescribed medication regimen and collaborating with a healthcare provider to adjust dosages as necessary is crucial for effective management. Medications help regulate blood sugar levels, but they work best when combined with lifestyle changes.

Regular monitoring of blood glucose levels provides valuable feedback on how well the management strategies are working. Using a glucometer to check blood sugar multiple times a day allows individuals to make informed decisions about their diet, exercise, and medication. This constant monitoring helps in making timely adjustments to maintain optimal blood sugar control and reduce the risk of complications associated with diabetes.

Blood Sugar Control During Pregnancy

Pregnancy presents distinct challenges for managing blood sugar levels, especially for women with gestational diabetes or pre-existing diabetes. Effective blood sugar control is vital for the well-being of both the mother and the baby.

Dietary Adjustments

A balanced diet is crucial during pregnancy to maintain stable blood sugar levels. Women should prioritize a diet rich in fruits, vegetables, lean proteins, and whole grains. These foods provide essential nutrients while helping to regulate blood sugar. Eating smaller, more frequent meals throughout the day can also aid in keeping blood sugar levels consistent. It's important to avoid sugary foods and drinks, as these can cause rapid spikes in blood glucose levels.

Physical Activity

Regular physical activity is beneficial for managing blood sugar levels during pregnancy, provided it's done safely. Low-impact exercises such as walking or swimming can be effective in regulating blood glucose levels and improving overall health. However, it's important to consult with a healthcare provider before starting any new exercise regimen to ensure it is safe and appropriate for the individual's specific condition.

Blood Glucose Monitoring

Frequent monitoring of blood glucose levels is essential for pregnant women with diabetes. Blood sugar levels may need to be checked multiple times a day to ensure they remain within the target range set by a healthcare provider. This monitoring helps in making necessary adjustments to insulin or medication dosages, ensuring that both the mother and the baby remain healthy.

Healthcare Provider Monitoring

Healthcare providers play a critical role in managing diabetes during pregnancy. They will closely monitor the health of both the mother and the baby throughout the pregnancy. This may involve additional tests and assessments to ensure blood sugar levels are well-controlled and to check for any potential complications. Regular check-ups are essential for making timely adjustments to the management plan and for ensuring that any issues are addressed promptly.

Blood Sugar Management For Athletes

For athletes, effective blood sugar management is crucial for sustaining energy, optimizing performance, and ensuring overall health. This involves a strategic approach to nutrition, exercise, and monitoring to maintain stable blood glucose levels.

Pre-Exercise Nutrition

Before exercise, it is essential to consume a well-balanced meal or snack. Aim to eat 1-3 hours prior to your workout, focusing on a combination of carbohydrates, proteins, and fats. Carbohydrates provide immediate energy, proteins support muscle repair, and fats offer sustained fuel. This approach helps in maintaining stable blood sugar levels and ensures that you have the energy needed for your workout. For example, a meal could include whole grains, lean protein, and a small amount of healthy fat.

Monitoring Blood Sugar

Monitoring blood sugar levels is key for managing fluctuations due to exercise. Checking blood glucose levels before starting your workout helps determine if they are in a safe range. Post-exercise monitoring is equally important as exercise can cause significant changes in blood sugar. Adjustments can be made based on these readings to maintain balance.

During Exercise

During extended or high-intensity exercise, athletes might experience drops in blood sugar levels. To counteract this, quick sources of carbohydrates are essential. Sports drinks, gels, and snacks designed for athletic performance can provide rapid glucose replenishment. It's beneficial to have these on hand, particularly for activities lasting over an hour or during high-intensity workouts.

Post-Exercise Recovery

After exercising, refueling is crucial. A balanced post-exercise meal should include carbohydrates and proteins to replenish glycogen stores and support muscle recovery. Carbohydrates help in restoring energy levels, while proteins are vital for repairing muscle tissues. For instance, a recovery snack might consist of a smoothie with fruit and protein powder or a whole-grain sandwich with lean protein.

Special Considerations for Athletes with Diabetes

Athletes with diabetes need to take additional steps to manage their blood sugar. Collaborating with a healthcare provider or sports nutritionist is recommended to create a personalized plan. This plan should account for the intensity, duration, and type of exercise to optimize both performance and health. Adjustments in insulin or medication may be necessary, and continuous monitoring can help prevent any adverse effects.

Considerations For Older Adults

As individuals age, their bodies undergo various changes that can significantly impact blood sugar management. These changes include decreased insulin sensitivity, a slower metabolism, and alterations in physical activity levels, all of which contribute to potential challenges in maintaining optimal blood sugar control.

One of the primary considerations for older adults is adapting their diet to meet shifting metabolic needs. A balanced diet becomes crucial, emphasizing foods rich in fiber, lean proteins, and healthy fats while minimizing processed foods and sugars. Portion control and meal timing also play pivotal roles in managing blood sugar levels effectively. Older adults should aim for consistent meal times and balanced portions to help stabilize glucose levels throughout the day.

Physical activity remains essential for maintaining overall health and managing blood sugar. However, exercise routines should be adjusted to accommodate individual capabilities and health conditions. Activities such as walking, gentle stretching, and strength training are particularly beneficial as they help preserve muscle mass, improve insulin sensitivity, and enhance overall mobility. It's important for older adults to engage in regular, moderate exercise that is safe and enjoyable to ensure long-term adherence and health benefits.

Regular monitoring of blood sugar levels is critical for detecting any fluctuations that may necessitate adjustments in diet, exercise, or medication. Healthcare providers recommend regular check-ups to assess overall health and modify treatment plans as needed to maintain stable blood sugar levels.

Managing medications can become more complex with age, especially when dealing with multiple health conditions or medications. Older adults should regularly review their medication regimen with healthcare providers to ensure that treatments effectively manage blood sugar levels without adverse interactions or side effects.

CHAPTER TEN

LONG-TERM SUCCESS

Maintaining Your Blood Sugar Diet

Maintaining a blood sugar diet over the long term requires embracing it as a lifestyle change rather than a temporary solution. Consistency is crucial for success. Adhering to the dietary guidelines you've established, such as monitoring carbohydrate intake, opting for whole foods, and ensuring balanced meals with adequate protein, healthy fats, and fiber, is fundamental. Staying hydrated and steering clear of excessive sugar and processed foods will also support your goals.

Meal planning is a valuable strategy to simplify adherence to your diet. By preparing meals ahead of time, you can save precious time and reduce the likelihood of making hasty, less nutritious food choices. Meal prepping helps you stick to your dietary plan by providing convenient, healthy options that align with your nutritional needs. Keep a selection of healthy snacks readily available to combat cravings and ensure you're prepared when hunger arises.

Regularly evaluating your dietary approach and making necessary adjustments is also important. Monitoring how your body responds to different foods and portion sizes can help you fine-tune your diet for optimal results. Experimenting with new foods and recipes can keep your meals exciting and enjoyable, preventing the diet from feeling monotonous or restrictive.

The goal is to integrate your blood sugar diet seamlessly into your daily routine. This approach helps in establishing sustainable eating habits that support long-term health and well-being. Remember, the aim is to create a balanced and manageable diet plan that becomes a natural part of your lifestyle, rather than viewing it as a temporary or restrictive regimen.

Tracking Your Progress

Tracking your progress is an essential part of any dietary regimen, especially if you're managing a condition like diabetes. Understanding how well your diet is working involves more than just monitoring your food intake; it requires a comprehensive approach to tracking various health metrics.

To begin with, maintaining a detailed food diary is highly recommended. This involves documenting everything you eat and drink, along with the timing of your meals and snacks. Record how each food item affects your blood sugar levels. This practice helps in identifying patterns and triggers that may influence your glucose readings. Numerous apps are available that can simplify this process, making it easier to log your meals and view your data in a structured format.

Regular monitoring of your blood sugar levels is another crucial aspect of tracking your progress. By checking your blood glucose at different times—such as before and after meals—you can observe how specific foods and dietary habits impact your levels. This information is invaluable for making necessary adjustments to your diet. If you're collaborating with a healthcare professional, sharing your tracking data with them is beneficial. They can analyze the information and provide expert guidance, helping you fine-tune your dietary choices for better outcomes.

Besides tracking food intake and blood sugar levels, it's important to monitor other aspects of your health. Pay attention to your energy levels, mood, and any symptoms you might experience. These factors can offer additional insights into the effectiveness of your diet. For instance, feeling more energetic or experiencing improved mood can be signs that your diet is having a positive impact, even if your blood sugar levels are not yet ideal.

Consistent tracking allows you to see trends and make informed adjustments. If certain foods or eating patterns lead to undesirable changes in your blood sugar or overall well-being, you can modify your approach accordingly. This proactive strategy helps in achieving better control over your health and ensures that your dietary plan is working effectively.

Adjusting Your Diet Over Time

As you advance in your health journey, it's crucial to recognize that your body's nutritional needs can evolve. This evolution may stem from a variety of factors including age, changes in physical activity levels, or shifts in overall health status. Adjusting your diet in response to these changes ensures that your nutritional intake remains optimal and supports your ongoing health objectives.

Understanding that dietary needs are not static can help you stay proactive about making necessary adjustments. For instance, as you age, your metabolism might slow down, or you might develop different health conditions that require specific dietary modifications. Likewise, changes in physical activity—whether you're becoming more active or scaling back—can also influence your nutritional requirements. It's essential to regularly evaluate your diet and make changes as needed.

If you start to notice that certain foods or meal patterns no longer serve your health goals effectively, it's time to explore alternatives. A common example is experiencing fluctuations in blood sugar levels after consuming certain foods. If you identify that a specific food causes an undesirable spike in blood sugar, consider replacing it with options that have a lower glycemic index. This change can help maintain more stable blood sugar levels and support better overall health.

Experimentation is key to finding what works best for you. Try different foods, adjust portion sizes, or modify meal timings to see how your body responds. Keep track of any changes in how you feel or any impact on health metrics. It's important to approach these adjustments thoughtfully and systematically.

Additionally, consulting with a healthcare provider or dietitian on a regular basis can provide valuable guidance. These professionals can help you reassess your dietary plan based on the latest evidence and your current health status. They can offer personalized recommendations and adjustments to ensure that your diet aligns with your evolving health needs and goals.

THE END

www.ingramcontent.com/pod-product-compliance
Lightning Source LLC
Chambersburg PA
CBHW070708250726